DON'T TOUCH YOUR FACE

YOUR FACE

poems from a pandemic

ANDREW WILLIAM SMITH
(ANDY SUNFROG)

Ordinary Books

DON'T TOUCH YOUR FACE: poems from a pandemic
by Andrew William Smith

The author considers all these words to be gifts. You are
welcome to copy or distribute these words in the context of non-
commercial personal sharing, as long as you provide credit.

For more information contact:
P.O. Box 1150
Cookeville, TN 38503
http://www.ordinaryspace.org/p/ordinary-books.html

Book and Cover design by Carolyn Oakley,
Luminous Moon Design, Boulder CO

Published by Ordinary Books, Cookeville, TN
ISBN: 978-0-9772258-3-5

First Edition: June 2021

These untitled, unnumbered poems were composed during the early days of the Covid crisis in the United States and distributed on many mornings via my Facebook feed. A year later, they still stand as unfiltered expressions and brief devotions for a world forever in crisis. They are meant to be read in order or out-of-order, one-at-a-time slowly or altogether in one sitting. Take them for what they are and simply enjoy.

A book, like life, is a collaborative endeavor. I am grateful as always to my family, especially my mother Barbara and my sweet spouse Jeannie. For editorial help with this book, we are grateful to Power Unit 17 Literary Services, and for design and helping us navigate our way to the finish line, we are grateful to Luminous Moon Design. Finally, a shout-out to my colleagues from the Ordinary Space fanzine, blog, and podcast projects, who agreed to have our "ordinary" name expand itself to include the launch of Ordinary Books. This is Ordinary Book #1 and hopefully the first of many publications under that banner.

Andrew/Sunfrog 2021
somewhere in middle "Tanasi," on the traditional land of the Cherokee people & the Yuchi tribe, also used or occupied by the Shawnee, Chickasaw, & Muscogee Creek people

panic shopping
it's what we do
pandemic fears
are coming for you

it's not only science or politics
when mixed with fear
just as long I remember not
to mix it with beer

just listen to the leaders
to make it all clear
Zuckerberg & Bezos will make a buck
off that same fear

don't tell me you get it because we don't understand
everyone's guessing right now &
would you like some of this sanitizer
to cover your hands

speaking of sanitizer
I think I'll make my own
out of all that booze they're drinking to
cope with pandemonium

the media measures the madness
in bloody darn clicks
until the
only ones

gathering outside the home
are music fans & 12-step alcoholics
who can't do online concerts or
online meetings anymore

don't hug don't kiss
don't touch your face
finally put all the masses
back in their proper place

don't touch your face
only makes me realize
that is all I ever want to do

don't go outside
are you crazy
get me gone right now

don't give into panic
on this off ramp of society
that is all i see

but when you are as
busy as me
slowing down might feel free

there is one thing
frightening but true
not talking to you

in particular but
all of us in
general

when somebody said
i wish people would
freak out about

climate change like
they are freaking
about the virus

this is one truth
less travel for
a period of time

is simply going
to be good
for the earth

in this season of
Lent & Easter
looking inward
waiting to see
what all this awareness of death
will bring to rebirth

my colleagues across
the country are

cancelling church
& frankly that

makes
sense

we have gone from
covid clueless to

covid cautious in
a few days &

from the fence I
have climbed

away from the middle
joined the ones playing fiddle

but as of now my
tiny church is planning
to meet

when they talk about
the days of the plague
don't be vague

hand sanitizer
lysol wipes
gloves & masks

if the grandchildren ask
are these liturgical objects
bless them & make them sacred

make your social distancing
as holy as the Lord's
boundary crossing to meet the Samaritan woman

even when the sudden
boundaries are
unreal

if this scary day is
anything it is not a

time for religious or political shame
for smarty smarmy gaslighting blame

no matter who you are

denomination
affiliation
atheist or monk
politics or none

to be alive is a
revolutionary act
to not be dead is
glorious resistance

so sing those dorky
church songs like
there is no tomorrow
because

there might be no tomorrow

universal imposed
mandatory sabbath
& if we get this right

the time is now for
cosmic jubilee
for the sake of the least

& vulnerable
give stuff away
forgive all debts

forget all sins
find & name
every silver lining

of unmistakable grace
quarantine hate
it's not too late

the world wakes up
from this fever dream
like this:

what are my feelings
who are my family
what is this world we

are fighting to save anyway
because the world in
my dream was pretty delicious yet

seeing all these preachers &
teachers & nurses & neighbors
just showing up for this thing

puts a knot in my throat
because we can do this
Lord loosen our lips

for every poem
every sermon
every song

every illegal hug
every secret social distance handshake
every makeshift underground restaurant

maybe we can reframe prohibition
to distill the moonshine of hope
be bootleggers of love

old-school outlaws of
human potential &
internet prophets of

unlimited grace

temple of toilet paper
conclave of cookies
bunker of light

ashram of anxiety
monastery of melody
isolation at night

shopping spree of solidarity
stress eating equality
virtual dance parties all day

ministry of internet
news channel of blues
memes of memory because

you are the you
that you were
meant to be

we are the ones
that we've
been waiting for

they won't
tell us
what is on the

other side
of this door

let's walk through

please just
stop showing me pictures
of intoxicated spring breakers

with judgy
eyerolls from your
immoral high ground

like you were never 21
never broke a rule
never got drunk

stop judging the
young adults
that you just handed

a world as messed up
& on fire as this
then made the only candidate

they liked into some
wild caricature
of evil before

turning around the
next day to start
implementing

some of those same
policies of generosity
before greed

just because—
you know—
the crisis

as if
the crisis
didn't start

in 1492
1776
1968
1945
1963
2016

stop judging the
teenagers & twenty-somethings
that have only

been out of potentially toxic
parental quarantine
a few years

because they want
to do the same
stupid things you did

at their age
please
just stop

hey
old people
like me

if i were 21 today
i would be up
to a lot worse

to more terrible
quarantine-defying
subversive mischief

than just going
to the beach
& getting drunk

covid code
crazy mode
getting old

shelter in place
voluntary quarantine
sleep but no dream

stress breathing is not
the same as
dying of disease

chocolate
cold shower
not another tornado warning

no longer say
keep it real
just keep it surreal

see two black crows
camped on your lawn
is that an omen

it must be an omen
we are all going to die
let me ask an adept

for her best guess
better than the mess
in my own head

but time for a nap
time for bed
we are all still

gonna end up dead
if not today
some day

retreat not defeat
you cannot eat
the stock market

there i said it
money man
get another plan

Jesus has such low
standards to identify with
people like us

but Chinese pollution
Italian canals
fewer cars on the road

so maybe
the wild earth
will still sustains us

thank us for
less pollution
cleaner water

maybe mother
nature is both forgiving
& saying heck to you

sad modernity
poison industry
the earth itself is

finally winning
nonrenewable diet
finally thinning

time is squishy
what day is it
the concept of time

we are missing
yet
you are made for this

wild shaman
kind pastor
good witch

spiritual antennae
on fire for a
situation this dire

don't itch
your
face

this is
no time
no place

to panic so
let's all panic
& eat organic

drink great gulps
from the Gatorade
of God's grace

dance in the rainfall
as mysterious mercy
fills this beautiful place

getting
dressed at 5am
but

there is
no place
to go

do you
suffer
from

anxiety
depression
PTSD

or could it be
addiction &
ADHD

last night we went
to bed at 9pm
got up at 11pm

watched late
night shows
until 1am

because
no reason
you just don't

need to justify
anything anymore
at home

not
what you eat
or don't eat

watch or
don't watch
including my weight

no more
virtual hate
virtuous play

"i am doing my
pandemic better
than your pandemic"

nah
blah
blah

one person said
"it's not a snow day"
another

"it's not a vacation"
okay
chill people

america
is giving everybody
a paid or unpaid

sabbath
today is Saturday
when God

commanded us
not gave us the
menu option

but ordered our
workaholic
whatevers to

slow
the blank
down

to please
just
stop

so no shame to
take a day off
turn off

the surveillance
camera in your
soul

puhleez
people
i know you

hate it
when i
say it but

really
i mean it
this time

we are
powerless
over this &

acceptance
is
the key &

it is
what
it is

I don't know
what time zone
it is

where you are
but one thing is
this collective insomnia

where we have
the chance
to dream

out loud &
dream
awake

so perhaps
the new
world

is born
like
this

weird world
where
the mask

is the
symbol
of safety

its absence
shows every
stupid illusion

of everything
finally
fully

unmasked

my small neighborhood
just got
incredibly large

there are places
to travel
by foot

incredible details
of wildlife &
litter

an entire universe
outside my door
that we could call

the shire
the strange
reality

of walking
of just going
outside

to move leaves
dirt
compost

around the yard
there is so
much to do

inside your mind
when there is
nothing to do

cultivate maps
to foreign lands
like a child

first exploring
her magic
fractal brain

from this dystopia
of daily
disaster drumbeats

draw a deep
yoga breath
mute your phone

& find the secret
maps to lost
childhood utopias

around the block
under a fence
inside a dying tree

eating all
the quarantine
snacks

look how
fast the
belly is back

Oreos creamy
Oreos yes
every flavor

is united
like white
and black

Eating Oreos
like Diane diPrima
ate Oreos

she said Oreos
make you
fat &

to Diane &
all the cookie
monster poets

we will tip our
panic snacking
hats

don't want
to go
to party zero

yet nobody
understood it
was party zero

when
party zero
began

so that means
no parties
at all

no parties
now so life
might celebrate

later
later
alligator

nobody goes
to party zero
except everybody

goes to church
to Walmart
to every place

party zero is
any place
people are

where the
disease
might be

everywhere
is the disease
& the disease

is everywhere
& party zero
is just a symbol

of why everyone
is sick & why
nobody still

gets it
the part about
isolation

but everybody
gets it
sick that is

not so much
the economy
but the reality

is what we miss
when we skip
party zero

one nation
under
lockdown

with lysol &
rubber gloves
for all

don't ask
if we know
anybody

who
has
"it"

because
this is
everywhere

you get a
text
message

get a
phone
call

see a
shocking
status &

then you
know
that we

were
warning
you

like a parent
warns
the child

with their
fingers near the
hot stove

don't wait
for the
text

from a
friend or
family member

to fall
apart
& cry

weep often
cry again
then repeat

if you
have anyone
in your

inner circle
at home
that you

are allowed
to hug
hug them

forgive every
foolish fight
before bed

every night
hold them
let them go

some of us
come from
a tradition

where surrender
does not mean
defeat

shelter in place
learn that
new pace

not just
in case
just because

we are
where we
are

i get it
i am sorry
some of your

friends are
not taking
this situation

with sufficient
seriousness
you don't like

the term
staycation
you hate

bible verses
& funny memes
you want

everyone to
feel as
miserable

about this mess
as you do
we are sorry

you saw someone
going to the
non-essential

business you saw
some people
gathered in a

group you even
heard that there
were people at

the bar & I get
it you want to
judge these people

their intelligence
their morals
even the Christians

you hate that
they want to
have church

when most ministers
even are begging
them to stay home

i get it you think
anyone not as
stressed as you

is a just
a toxic optimist
a privileged pollyanna

i hear you
i am sorry
for my guilt

in this
my tornado
survivor's guilt

now pandemic
survivor's guilt
even our

geography
our gender race
& class

have something to
do with how
much we judge

the people who
share our gender
race or class

because middle class
white people shaming
other middle class

white people on
social media is how
we make revolution

not really
but i get it
because

we
are scared
too

& uncertain fear
prompts us to
say silly things

to say i am
better than you spiritually
more woke than you politically

even test &
tempt the rules
of the quarantine

see nobody asked
for this nobody
wanted this

but even this
is ripping up
every illusion

until we make
these media
rants into a

mirror of love
& loss & longing
where yes you

can be both
powerless &
empowered

at the same
freaking
time

some day you
will exhale &
remove the nail

from your heart
but until then
every freaking day

is just another
freaking day
to breathe

to rethink
to renew
to restart

just
wrong
it is all

just so scary
wrong & now
this

not another
obituary not
another death

grief &
denial &
not enough grief

what anger
what bargaining
what fear

please forgive me
for not
forgiving myself

or just forgive
me for that thing
i said or didn't say

catch your breath
from too
many storms

gasping
grasping &
multi-tasking

Jesus cried
Jesus ugly cried
then Jesus died

who are all
those people
not six feet

apart who
are they kidding
not six inches

pinch me
we must be
dreaming

the blue sky
flowers budding
all so deceptive

the mood is
springtime
but then it

isn't because
they are
going to

cancel Easter
not exactly
a thing we do

Easter is just
not that day at
that building

when we
celebrate
that other thing

resurrection though
are we even
allowed to say

it anew
across the chasm
between life

& death
heaven &
this time warp

did the earth
stop moving
this disease

is the enemy
we are allowed
to hate it

every day of
the last
three weeks

replay it
again &
again

until you
believe it
yourself

until you
lift an
arm through

the pain
because new
life still gains

a place past
stress-eating
chocolate eggs

& marshmallow
rabbits make the
sugar high last

not looking
for
Jesus

except
in the
present

not
the future or
the past

come Lord
Jesus
now

guilty as
in the insides
compared

to the outsides
& outside
is hell

my survivor's
guilt has
survivor's guilt

guilty for
not doing
enough

guilty for
doing too
much

guilty
for
living

guilty
for not
dying

guilty for
having a
good day

guilty for
going to
the store

then guilty
for internally
criticizing

every single
person at
the same store

for being
in the
store

during the
pandemic
but panic

shopping
is totally
essential, right

guilty to
wake up
in the middle

of the night
get up to
do your chores

but just
write poems &
make playlists

instead because
we need more
poems & playlists

to watch
this horror
show pass

forgiven
folks should
not feel

like crap
but some
folks are

just wired
like
that

i prayed
with someone
who has the virus

i prayed
with a health
care worker

who is
isolating
i will pray

with you
if you
ask

that seems
to be the
one thing

that helps
no i am
not one

who thinks
that praying
is instead

of science
medicine or
common sense

don't make me
also feel
guilty for that

tune in
tomorrow
with

another
strong
feeling

we will
be
back

Google
these
words

intubation
aerosolization
anthropocene

I don't want
to Google
how many

cruise ships
are stuck
at sea

Google will
now tell
you what

this pandemic
is doing
to me

while we
are preaching
sabbath

whether we
want it
or not

we are
not sleeping
or sleeping

too much
we have
stockpiled

too much
some don't
have enough

we are making
an easter basket
to give to

a stranger
which might
make us feel

better for
just an hour
about all

this present
danger
but then

as insomnia
fades to
actual morning

the birds
are singing
in the yard

how did
i write so
many darn

pandemic poems
but for the birds
are like the bard

holy
headphones
of hope

my early
morning
meditation

has been
music
maybe podcasts

maybe a
sermon
or even

informative
YouTube
here and there

so on a
dare to
myself

this morning
i drank
in nothing

but silence
so incredible
the sound

of silence
which of
course

makes
me want
to listen to

that haunting
song
right now

so many
little wows
from the

inner
landscape
this is

how we
survive
isolation

with daily
meditation
transformation

but that silence
I had avoided
even alone

is suddenly
so sublime
so sweet

we can
bend our
brains

that is
so
neat

& sure like
that one
meme

said that on
some days
setting a schedule

would be
nice but
some days

time falls
apart in
glorious

casual
unstructured
disarray

in praise
of all
the useless

unnecessary
nonessential
things

in praise
of these
cookies

in praise
of this
collage

in praise
of paint
of poetry

of compost
of cats
of cardboard fires

in praise of crazy
posts on
Twitter

Facebook
Instagram
even email

in praise of
unnecessary
nonessential

snacks
cat pictures
music videos

did I mention
cats
we don't have

one nonessential
cat or bird
or rabbit

but we have
our nonessential
frivolous loves

stuck at home
to do our
nonessential

things
that make
the essential

facts of this
global freakout
more bearable

don't touch
your
face

shelter
in
place

what is
this
pace

don't touch
your
face

shelter
in
place

in this
weird
place

one minute
i am reading
then writing

about the
total collapse
of everything

society
as we
know it

has a
few weeks
few months

at best
before
it all

falls
completely
apart

this is
the day
that your

utopias
dystopias
& Bibles

been
warning you
about

sure some
good can
come from

this but
not without
lots of bad

the dark
day of
the Lord

is here
& there
ain't

nothing
we can
do about it

morgue
mass grave
mass panic

shortages
soup lines
riots

empty churches
empty schools
overflowing hospitals

kiss
the whole
modern

whatever
goodbye
forever

then i
took a
nice walk

in my
sunny
neighborhood

i have
never seen
so many

of my
neighbors
before

each in their
own yard
playing

grilling
drinking
trampoline

sweet
american
pastoral narcotic

so maybe
the end
isn't here

just yet
at least not
on this

early
April
Friday

can't sleep
for how
many nights

now can't
stop
sleeping

can't
stop
dreaming

& of course
it is a
quarantine dream

dream as quarantine
dream about quarantine
wait not

really it is
a pandemic dream
not a dream

but a nightmare &
everyone is sick
& not six feet apart

everyone is together
playing music
but they are dying

we are dying
I am dying
I am

awake now
wow
I slept in

get me
some darn
coffee fast

wildfires
hurricanes
floods

blizzards
tornadoes
thunderstorms

glaciers
mountains
oceans

now this
freaking
pandemic

stop
stop
just stop

so today
they said
a tiger

not the
Tiger King
but an

actual freaking
tiger like
at the zoo

yes a
tiger has
the virus

so no
we don't
need no

simplistic
narrative
about nature

fighting back
yet nature
is fighting

yet just
stop
please just

stop
overthinking
stop pretending

stop saying
we know
what we don't know

because we
don't know
much

so please
for a moment
stop because we

are required
to anyways so
please listen

breathe deep
pay attention
then

stop
some
more

check
on your
saints

check on
them
now

by telephone
by email
by USPS

whatever
it
takes

just check
on them
living saints

then
namecheck
some now

Diane diPrima
Gary Snyder
Lawrence Ferlinghetti

living
Beat
royalty

Anne Waldman
Wendell Berry
Coleman Barks

listen
to
them

see I just found
out that
Ernesto Cardenal

is dead had
died earlier in
the year

but with
everything
going on

I found
out
late

so please
if you have
the chance

just check
on your
saints

squishy time
softened from
weird wide

not so slow
sleeping more
learning new

time so it
sped back up
suddenly abnormal

is getting normal
not sure we
like this then

we go out for
supplies &
what's this

I am thanking
every single
worker that

I meet just
for working
at a retail store

thank you
for being here
some smile

sometimes you
can see
the smile

even under
the mask
through the

eyes are
on us
yes us

are we
mostly
sort of

staying home
except these
store runs

spaced out
by days
then what is

this is
Walmart
I was the

kind of
person who
doesn't like

Walmart &
now suddenly
it's like

Walmart
is the most
amazing place

you have
ever seen
really not

ironic or
kidding
this weird

way has
made me
love WalMart

maybe that
is a side effect
hopefully not

the plan
all
along

gravel road
back of
the hollow

with trees & breeze
& dogs & logs &
guinea fowl

we brought
an Easter
basket

to an old
woman
who had lived

on that land
for years & years
& years

our brief moment
at a distance
could not capture

the spirit of
her small frame
or giant smile

but she did
have one thing
to say

when we
asked about
the storm of

two Sundays
past which
she said

skipped over
her house
her neighbors not

so lucky she
had one thing
to say about that

she said her
father always
used to tell her

to look out
for the Easter
storm & that

maybe that last
one was this
year's Easter storm

but now here we are
it is Easter &
it is raining hard

rainy Easter afternoon
the wife & me sit
she is sewing

& I am typing
& we are listening
to jazz but we

never listen to
jazz yet right now
it is Duke Ellington

because I had been reading
The Seven Storey Mountain
by Merton & young Merton

was always listening to blues
& jazz especially Ellington
so here we are on Easter

listening to Ellington like
80 some years after Merton was
listening to Ellington

typing sewing listening
to jazz & watching the
Easter rain rain rain

outside our window
& this Easter in the
year of the plague it

would rain & they would
be calling for more
bad storms just like the

woman at the back of the
hollow with the guinea fowl
said beware of the Easter

storms now it is Sunday
& we are listening to jazz
& typing & sewing & I am

worrying about the
Easter storms that
might come tonight

we are praying &
prepared but not assured
about anything

not assured about
sunshine on Easter
not assured about

the outcome of this
plague or even the
health of our loved

ones just knowing
a handful of things
like the tomb is

empty the cake is
sweet the coffee is
strong we are listening

to jazz & sewing &
typing & waiting out
another Easter storm

not long ago
I read the books
watched the YouTube

learned that trees
can talk
that is right trees

communicate with
each other through
their roots

so last night when
on my proverbial
knees I tried to

talk to the trees
the dozens &
dozens of trees

in my yard &
neighboring yards
I asked the trees

to keep their
roots rooted
even with branches

swaying
bending in
the wild wind

yes I asked the
trees from
my knees

to stay rooted
deep deep in
this tiny patch

of Tennessee earth
no trees uprooted
no trees causing harm

I pray to God
but times like now
I talk to trees

why not
with so many
storms so much

unknown it is
okay if you talk
to trees too

what's your
pandemic
paradigm

struck
by perfect
Pauline light

knocked from
your collective ego
economic high horse

into a mystical
swirl of redeemed
ecological meaning or

maybe it is
just your
perspective

just your
privilege
to see a

silver lining
in this
touch of grey

even in sober
moderation
we want a good story

about a decent
society giving up
its addiction

to bad things
like bad pollution
bad power-hungry stuff

we need this to
stop everything to
mean something

more than
mere human
ugly mess

we confess
magical thinking
virtue signaling

some kind
of majestic
moral narrative

not this
nihilistic now
with weird tails

wagging no
nice nagging
no more tales

snagging in
alarmist all
red flagging

I got mad
because of
something that

I read on
the Internet
I know that

never happens
to anyone else
not

not going to lie
my feelings are
bunched up drawers

not going to reply
not this thread
social media fighting

until all our
brains are dead
we are judge

judge judge
judge & jury
& sentencing too

there is nothing
wrong with me
the problem is

always you
you are too
right wing or

you are too
left wing or
too religious

or too atheist
or too you & a
world where

everyone agrees
with me would
be so perfect

not like
I would stop
complaining

about Trump
Obama Bush
or Clinton if

I was king
all the peace
wealth & justice

I would bring
with my free market
socialism capitalism

hippy dippy
perfect year-round
festival for all

universal basic
Twitter feed
every need

met because
everyone thinks
that I am

the king
of the whole
freaking Internet

do not
start to
Google all

the reasons
for this
just don't

even the
science theories
are scary

just because
they call
it guano

doesn't mean
it's not gross
or that we are all

goners yeah
if you had
asked me

for my ideas
for what would
take down

the world what
would we
say maybe

a terror bomb
climate change
oil spill

who knows
but bat poop
really has

it come
to this thing
maybe don't

thank nature or
blame nature
but go wow

we humans are
powerless
over bat poop

I love Jesus & all
but there is
that time in

everyone's quarantine
where you seriously
consider asking an

Oreo cookie to be
your personal
Lord & Savior

now as
a recovered addict
I walk that

stuff back because
I know where
it takes me

but just to
tell on myself
the thought

crossed
my
mind

slow your roll
not so fast
what's the hurry

learn not
from the present
or the past

if you just
get out of town
to get on

the road
there seems
to be a panic

to just
open throttle
& go go go

but if we
are the ones
learning the new

art of pause
finding a new
cause in the

community alone
making sense
of our home

not just
Netflix & crafts
maybe garden this

or a little bit
of that & now
a new kind

of respect
for the power
of life

the reality
of death
the health

of our planet
more stuff you
cannot buy

& nobody can
buy anything if
we all go & die

just make it
mean something
any meaning

will do
we just want
stories to tell

our virtual
grandchildren
some day

when this
is over
what do you mean

we might never
be the same
the world will

look back with
sentimental fears
memorial tears

to the days
of new routines
entertainment fatigue

the virus
that could not
kill greed

there are many
days where i
need that extra

something just
to survive
the moment

let's not
shame or
blame game

true there is
so much to do
when there is

nothing you
can do
who who who

prays
plays
waits

don't hate me
for talking about
sunlight in the

moonlight
or for admitting
that I like

garlic
vinegar
sage

at my age
at this stage
after all this

rage
plague
don't be

so vague
we just want
to live for

one
more
day

didn't
believe
Buddha

couldn't
believe
the Bible

started to
believe
Huxley & Blake

doors of perception
road to excess
palace of wisdom

then Duncan Trusell
asked you on his podcast
about acronyms for God

when they
told me
"good orderly direction"

I thought
that sounds
boring

but this
"gift of desperation"
I get that

thanks
Anne Lamott
e.e. cummings

thanks for reminding
me that it was
not the good book

but a bad drunk
that finally led
me to Jesus

things I learned
or heard on
Zoom today

there are no
more regular
days like Monday

or dates like
today would be
the 28th

instead there are
just three days
yesterday today

tomorrow but
that was just
on one Zoom

room in the
morning but
then on a

different Zoom
in the afternoon
with pastor friends

I learned that
there are two
kinds of days

just Sunday
&
not Sunday

I learned
some more
amazing things

on Zoom
today that
I cannot say

but don't
let that get
in the way

of you telling
us about your
Zoom day

just five summers
ago I stood at the
base of some

Colorado mountains
walking around
with my headphones on

when the track
"Rocket Man" but
not the Elton John

one yet the My
Morning Jacket
version came on

& suddenly I
felt so incredibly
small a citizen

of great galaxies
& time felt so
incredibly brief

this quick sprint
through life
my few decades

a tiny click when
seen in cosmic terms
did you ever feel

so brief
so small
as that

well let me
tell you that
this pandemic

brings that feeling
back so fast
to stay

please just
get out of
our own way

we are so little
for such a little
gasp of now

everything is fragile
everything is fleeting
but this is not

some book of
Ecclesiastes
cynical pity pot

no not never
sad okay maybe
just a little sad

yet barely
because now
is forever &

we better
be freaking grateful
for that

fifteen years ago
this week I lost
my teaching job

let go at semester's
end without notice
just like that

eleven years ago
this weekend I lost
my best friend

alcohol which
was no longer
my friend &

was trying
to
kill me

so suddenly
i look back
to standing

on the edge
of a cliff with
my back against

the wall &
remember that
despite my privilege

I have some worry
some fear
some anxiety

in common with
those sleeping in
tents under bridges

with those looking
for work waiting
for checks standing

in line hoping
for some free food
& if I never forget

what it feels like
to be unemployed
to be a drunk

at the end
of his rope
I will never

forget what it
feels like to be
desperate enough

to let go
& desperate enough
to live

just like that
right on time
over here

they are open
speeding cars
biker bars

but not
unlike an
open wound

what is the hurry
wild without worry
they kill fear

with plexiglass
some masks
is the day of

the Lord here
this year
let's be clear

I want to be wrong
a different song
let it be over

next crisis please
but I am still
on my knees

forever changed
by a disease that
touched family

& friends &
is this how
it ends

just back to
business back
to before

just open
the door
on a definition

of freedom
that never
existed

multicolored bandana &
rubber gloves
seem normal now

all these cars
in such a hurry
that seems strange

where are we
going where
have we been

I don't know anything
I have no power
just live hour to hour

grateful for all
these books all
these movies

all this music
all this art but I
really got

freaked out when
the internet was
down for just

a few hours like
the internet is
some sacrament

big brother wires
up in my brain
but the Netflix

& the Hulu
the Audible too &
yes the Spotify

the breeze outside
anxiety subsides
suddenly okay

it took a hospital
chaplain to
tell me

that even
though her
clients could

not see her
smile that
they could still

see Jesus because
of—not in spite
of—the mask

in the hospital
the mask shows love
shows Christ or

if you prefer
plain ordinary
human love

get it please
this pandemic
is a trudge

a tortoise not
a hare so why
do you dare

hold a grudge
act like a
judge just because

some cover their face
hide my smile or
mischievous smirk

don't curse them
if they ask you
to put on that mask

don't hate them
kill them or call
them names because

they wear the
mask that shows
their love better

than any poem
or rant ever
could or would

after the test
not much changed
asymptomatic is a word

that we kept repeating
living in quarantine
separate in the same house

from the one you love
from the work you love
from the friends but not

from the news
from the bad news
from the good news

as pandemic gives
way to protest
the cases still surge

we resist that strange urge
to pretend everything
is back to normal

when we now wonder
if it will
ever be

normal again
if it was normal then
it will be abnormal when

the endless
summer
treadmill

of work & die
the political lie of
open the schools

like we never knew
the sadistic fate of
selfish educated fools